# Home Exercise Guide Made Simple for Beginners

## Creating a Comfortable Exercise Space

By

Brice Clayton

# Table of Contents


CHAPTER 1.................................................6

Introduction ..............................................6

1.1 Why Exercise at Home? ...............6

1.2 Setting Realistic Goals..................9

CHAPTER 2...............................................13

Getting Started ........................................13

2.1 Creating a Comfortable Exercise Space.......................................................13

2.2 Necessary Equipment and Gear..15

2.3 Warm-up and Cool-down Routines .................................................................18

CHAPTER 3...............................................21

Understanding Exercise Basics ............21

3.1 Types of Exercises (Cardio, Strength, Flexibility)......................21

3.2 Proper Form and Technique .......24

3.3 Breathing and Posture.................26

CHAPTER 4...............................................28

Building Your Home Workout Routine
................................................................28

4.1 Setting a Schedule.......................28

4.2 Choosing the Right Exercises.....30

4.3 Progression and Adaptation........32

CHAPTER 5..................................35

Cardiovascular Exercises.................35

5.1 Jumping Jacks............................35

5.2 High Knees................................37

5.3 Jump Rope.................................38

5.4 Dancing for Fitness....................40

CHAPTER 6..................................42

Strength Training.............................42

6.1 Bodyweight Exercises (Push-ups, Squats, Planks)...................................42

6.2 Using Household Items as Weights
................................................................45

6.3 Resistance Band Workouts.........46

CHAPTER 7..................................49

Flexibility and Mobility....................49

7.1 Stretching Exercises....................49

7.2 Yoga and Pilates for Beginners ..51

7.3 Foam Rolling Techniques...........53

CHAPTER 8.............................................56

Staying Motivated ...............................56

8.1 Setting and Tracking Goals.........56

8.2 Finding Support and
Accountability.....................................58

8.3 Overcoming Common Challenges
...............................................................61

CHAPTER 9.............................................63

Safety and Injury Prevention................63

9.1 Listening to Your Body ..............63

9.2 Common Exercise Mistakes to
Avoid ...................................................65

9.3 Dealing with Injuries .................68

CHAPTER 10...........................................70

Nutrition and Recovery .......................70

10.1 Fueling Your Body ...................70

10.2 Post-Workout Nutrition ...........72

10.3 Rest and Recovery ....................74

CHAPTER 11.......................................77

Tracking Your Progress ......................77

11.1 Keeping a Workout Journal ......77

11.2 Measuring Success....................79

# CHAPTER 1

# Introduction

## 1.1 Why Exercise at Home?

Exercising at home has gained significant popularity over recent years, and for a multitude of compelling reasons. For beginners, in particular, the concept of home workouts provides an inviting and accessible entry point into the world of fitness. Here are several key reasons why one might choose to exercise at home:

1. **Convenience**: One of the most prominent advantages of home workouts is the unparalleled convenience they offer. You're not bound by the constraints of gym hours or long commutes.

You can exercise at any time
that suits your schedule,
making it easier to establish a
consistent routine.

2. **Privacy**: For many beginners,
   the idea of working out in a
   crowded gym can be
   intimidating. Exercising at
   home provides a private and
   comfortable setting where you
   can build confidence and focus
   on your fitness journey without
   any self-consciousness.

3. **Cost-Effective**: Gym
   memberships and fitness
   classes can be expensive. Home
   workouts eliminate the need for
   these recurring expenses,
   making fitness more affordable,
   especially for those just
   starting.

4. **Customization**: Exercising at home allows you to tailor your workouts to your specific goals, preferences, and comfort level. You can choose exercises that align with your interests and adapt routines as you progress.

5. **Minimal Equipment**: While you can invest in equipment, many effective home workouts can be done with little to no equipment. This makes it accessible for individuals with limited space or budget.

6. **Family and Community**: Home workouts can be a great way to involve family members or create a sense of community with others who share similar fitness goals. It's an excellent way to encourage family bonding and mutual support.

7. **Health and Safety**: Especially relevant during times of public health concerns, exercising at home minimizes exposure to crowded spaces and provides a more controlled and hygienic environment.

In essence, exercising at home offers a plethora of benefits that can be especially enticing for beginners. It eliminates many of the common barriers to starting a fitness routine and provides a platform for establishing a strong foundation for a healthier lifestyle.

## 1.2 Setting Realistic Goals

Setting realistic goals is an essential step for anyone embarking on a fitness journey, especially beginners. Goals serve as the guiding light, motivating and directing your efforts. However, setting the right kind of goals is crucial to ensure that they are achievable and sustainable. Here's why this aspect is vital:

1. **Motivation**: Realistic goals provide motivation. They give you a reason to get up and work out each day. When you see progress toward your goals, it reinforces your commitment to exercise.

2. **Sustainability**: Unrealistic goals can lead to frustration and burnout. By setting achievable milestones, you're more likely to stick with your workout routine in the long term.

3. **Progress Tracking**: Realistic goals are measurable and allow you to track your progress. This

tracking is essential for making necessary adjustments and celebrating your achievements.

4. **Preventing Injury**: Unrealistic goals can lead to overtraining and increased risk of injury. Realistic goals allow you to push yourself within safe limits, avoiding potential setbacks.

5. **Building Confidence**: Achieving smaller, realistic goals builds confidence. As a beginner, these small victories are invaluable for your self-esteem and commitment to your fitness journey.

6. **Adaptability**: Realistic goals are flexible and can adapt to your changing circumstances or abilities. They allow you to

pivot and modify your plan as
needed.

# CHAPTER 2

# Getting Started

## 2.1 Creating a Comfortable Exercise Space

Creating a comfortable exercise space at home is fundamental to ensure a positive and effective workout experience. Here's why this step is significant and how to go about it:

- **Motivation and Environment**: Your exercise space should be inviting and motivate you to work out. A clutter-free, well-lit area can be more inspiring than a chaotic or dim space. Personalize it with motivating quotes, music, or anything that makes you feel energized.

- **Safety**: Ensure that your exercise area is free of hazards. Clear away objects that could cause accidents or obstruct your movements. Providing a safe environment is crucial, especially if you're a beginner.

- **Space Considerations**: While you don't need a large area, make sure you have enough room to perform various exercises comfortably. Different workouts may require different amounts of space, so plan accordingly.

- **Ventilation**: A well-ventilated space is essential to prevent overheating and discomfort during workouts. Proper airflow can also improve your overall exercise experience.

- **Privacy**: If you're concerned about privacy, choose a space where you can exercise without feeling self-conscious or exposed. This can help you focus on your routine without distractions.

Your exercise space can evolve over time as you become more experienced and dedicated to your workouts. The initial setup is important, but you can always make improvements as you go.

## 2.2 Necessary Equipment and Gear

One of the great advantages of home exercise is that it can be done with minimal or no equipment. This accessibility makes it an attractive option for beginners. Here's what you need to know about equipment and gear:

- **Bodyweight Exercises**: Many effective workouts can be performed using your body weight alone. Exercises like push-ups, squats, lunges, and planks are excellent choices for beginners. They help build strength and flexibility without requiring any equipment.

- **Basic Equipment**: While optional, some basic equipment can enhance your workouts. Items like a yoga mat, resistance bands, and dumbbells (if you have them) can add variety and intensity to your routines. However, they are not essential for starting out.

- **Footwear and Clothing**: Wear comfortable, breathable clothing that allows you to move freely. The right footwear is essential; opt for shoes that provide adequate support and stability for the types of exercises you'll be doing.

- **Safety Gear**: If you have specific health concerns or are recovering from an injury, consult a healthcare professional about any necessary safety gear. For example, a knee brace or wrist support may be beneficial in certain cases.

The most important aspect of equipment and gear for beginners is starting with what you have and gradually adding items as your fitness journey progresses. You don't need an extensive collection of gear to begin your home workouts; simplicity can be highly effective.

## 2.3 Warm-up and Cool-down Routines

Warm-up and cool-down routines are often overlooked, but they are critical for a safe and effective workout. Here's why they matter and how to incorporate them into your home exercise routine:

- **Warm-up Benefits**: A proper warm-up prepares your body for exercise by increasing your heart rate, blood flow to muscles, and joint mobility. It helps prevent injuries and prepares your mind for the workout ahead.

- **Warm-up Components**: A warm-up should include light cardio, such as jumping jacks or jogging in place, followed by dynamic stretches to loosen up your muscles. This can last around 5-10 minutes.

- **Cool-down Benefits**: The cool-down is essential to gradually reduce your heart rate and relax your muscles after a workout. It can prevent muscle soreness and stiffness and promote flexibility.

- **Cool-down Components**: Cool-down exercises include static stretches that you hold for 15-30 seconds per muscle group. Focus on areas you worked during your workout. This phase also lasts about 5-10 minutes.

Incorporating warm-up and cool-down routines into your home exercise regimen is non-negotiable. These routines ensure you're physically and mentally prepared for your workout and help your body recover afterward. Skipping them can increase the risk of injury and hinder your progress.

# CHAPTER 3

# Understanding Exercise Basics

## 3.1 Types of Exercises (Cardio, Strength, Flexibility)

Understanding the different types of exercises is fundamental for creating a well-rounded fitness routine that addresses various aspects of physical health. Here's an overview of these exercise categories and their importance:

- **Cardiovascular Exercises (Cardio)**: Cardio exercises are designed to elevate your heart rate, improve cardiovascular health, and burn calories. They include activities like jogging, jumping jacks, cycling, and dancing. Cardio workouts increase endurance, help with weight management, and are vital for heart health.

- **Strength Training Exercises**: Strength training focuses on building muscle strength and endurance. It typically involves resistance exercises using your body weight, free weights, or resistance bands. Examples include push-ups, squats, and dumbbell curls. Strength training not only enhances physical strength but also supports bone health and metabolism.

- **Flexibility Exercises**: Flexibility exercises, such as

stretching and yoga, aim to improve the range of motion of your joints and reduce muscle tension. Regular flexibility work can enhance posture, reduce the risk of injury, and promote relaxation and stress relief.

- **Balancing the Types of Exercises**: A well-rounded fitness routine should include elements from all three categories: cardio, strength, and flexibility. The specific balance will depend on your goals, fitness level, and personal preferences. Beginners may start with a balanced mix and adjust over time as they progress.

## 3.2 Proper Form and Technique

Proper form and technique are critical for performing exercises safely and effectively. Understanding and practicing good form can help prevent injuries and ensure that you're targeting the right muscle groups. Here's why this aspect is crucial:

- **Injury Prevention**: Using correct form reduces the risk of strains, sprains, and other exercise-related injuries. It ensures that your body is moving in a biomechanically efficient manner.

- **Targeted Muscle Engagement**: Proper form ensures that you're engaging the intended muscle groups, maximizing the benefits of each exercise.

- **Better Results**: Correct technique leads to more effective workouts. You'll see faster progress and achieve your fitness goals more efficiently.

- **Mind-Body Connection**: Paying attention to form encourages a mind-body connection. You become more aware of how your body moves and feels during exercise.

- **Form Troubleshooting**: Beginners should consider working with a fitness professional or using instructional videos to learn and practice proper form. Feedback and guidance can be invaluable.

## 3.3 Breathing and Posture

Breathing and posture are often overlooked aspects of exercise, yet they play a crucial role in ensuring a safe and effective workout:

- **Breathing**: Proper breathing during exercise provides your muscles with the oxygen they need. For many exercises, exhale during the effort (e.g., when lifting weights) and inhale during the release. Maintaining a steady breathing rhythm is important for endurance and energy.

- **Posture**: Correct posture ensures that your body is aligned in a way that minimizes strain and supports good form. It's especially important during strength and flexibility exercises. Poor posture can lead

to muscle imbalances and
discomfort.

- **Alignment and Balance**: Pay
  attention to alignment,
  particularly in exercises
  involving the spine, hips, and
  shoulders. Maintaining balance
  and alignment helps prevent
  injuries and promotes better
  overall body mechanics.

# CHAPTER 4

# Building Your Home Workout Routine

## 4.1 Setting a Schedule

Establishing a workout schedule is a fundamental step in maintaining consistency and making exercise a habit. Here's why scheduling matters and some tips on setting one:

- **Consistency**: Having a set schedule helps you stay consistent with your workouts. It creates a routine that makes it easier to prioritize exercise.

- **Accountability**: A schedule can be a form of accountability. When you plan and allocate specific times for exercise, you're more likely to follow through.

- **Time Management**: Scheduling allows you to manage your time effectively. You can plan your workouts around other commitments and responsibilities.

- **Goal Alignment**: Your schedule should align with your fitness goals. For instance, if your goal is to build strength, you might have different workout days compared to someone aiming for cardiovascular fitness.

- **Realistic Expectations**: Be realistic about the time you can commit. Start with a manageable schedule and gradually increase workout frequency as you become more comfortable.

- **Flexibility**: While schedules are essential, allow for flexibility. Life can be unpredictable, so it's okay to adjust your workout days and times when necessary.

## 4.2 Choosing the Right Exercises

Selecting the right exercises for your home workout routine is crucial for achieving your fitness goals. Here's how to choose the exercises that best suit you:

- **Goal-Oriented**: Choose exercises that align with your specific fitness goals. For instance, if you want to

improve your cardiovascular
health, incorporate cardio
exercises. If strength is your
aim, focus on strength training
exercises.

- **Variety**: Include a variety of
exercises to work different
muscle groups and prevent
boredom. A well-rounded
routine not only promotes
overall fitness but also keeps
you engaged.

- **Progression**: Consider
exercises that can be modified
or progressed over time. This
allows you to continually
challenge yourself as you
become fitter. For example, you
can start with basic push-ups
and work towards more
challenging variations.

- **Enjoyment**: Select exercises that you enjoy. If you like an activity, you're more likely to stick with it. Experiment with different workouts to find what you love.

- **Safety**: Ensure that the exercises you choose are safe and appropriate for your fitness level. If you're uncertain, seek guidance from a fitness professional.

## 4.3 Progression and Adaptation

Progression and adaptation are essential for ongoing success and continuous improvement in your fitness journey. Here's why they matter and how to implement them:

- **Progressive Overload**: To see progress, gradually increase the intensity, duration, or complexity of your workouts. This could mean adding more weight, increasing repetitions, or shortening rest periods.

- **Listening to Your Body**: Pay attention to how your body responds to your workouts. If you experience pain or discomfort, it may be time to adapt your routine or seek guidance.

- **Periodization**: Consider periodization, which involves dividing your training into cycles, each with a specific focus. This prevents plateaus and keeps your workouts fresh.

- **Recovery**: Don't forget the importance of rest and recovery. Your body needs time to repair and grow stronger. Schedule rest days into your routine and allow for adequate sleep.

- **Adaptation to Goals**: As your fitness goals evolve, so should your workout routine. If your objectives change, adjust your exercises and schedule accordingly.

# CHAPTER 5

# Cardiovascular Exercises

## 5.1 Jumping Jacks

Jumping jacks are a classic and effective cardiovascular exercise that can be done without any equipment. Here's why they're beneficial and how to perform them:

- **Benefits**:

    - Improves cardiovascular fitness.

    - Engages multiple muscle groups, including legs, arms, and core.

- Enhances coordination and agility.

- Can be easily modified for different fitness levels.

- **How to Do Jumping Jacks:**

1.     Stand with your feet together and arms at your sides.

2.     Jump your feet out to the sides while raising your arms overhead.

3.     Jump back to the starting position with your feet together and arms at your sides.

4.     Repeat in a continuous, rhythmic motion.

## 5.2 High Knees

High knees are another effective cardio exercise that also improves lower body strength. Here's why they're valuable and how to perform them:

- **Benefits**:

  - Elevates heart rate and boosts cardiovascular fitness.

  - Strengthens leg muscles, including quadriceps and hip flexors.

  - Enhances balance and coordination.

  - Helps improve running form and speed.

- **How to Do High Knees**:

1.    Stand with your feet hip-width apart.

2.    Lift one knee as high as possible while bringing the opposite arm up.

3.    Quickly switch to the other knee and arm.

4.    Keep alternating knees in a marching or running motion

## 5.3 Jump Rope

Jumping rope is a classic cardiovascular exercise that requires minimal equipment and provides an effective full-body workout. Here's why it's a great choice and how to do it:

- **Benefits**:

- Elevates heart rate and enhances cardiovascular endurance.

- Engages leg muscles and core.

- Improves coordination and agility.

- Burns a significant number of calories in a short time.

- **How to Jump Rope**:

1.     Stand with your feet together and hold the jump rope handles in each hand.

2.     Swing the rope over your head and jump over it as it passes under your feet.

3.     Keep a steady rhythm and land softly on the balls of your feet.

## 5.4 Dancing for Fitness

Dancing for fitness is a fun and dynamic way to get your heart rate up while enjoying music and movement. Here's why it's a great option for cardiovascular exercise:

- **Benefits**:

    - Elevates heart rate and improves cardiovascular fitness.

    - Enhances coordination, balance, and rhythm.

    - Provides a full-body workout.

    - Boosts mood and reduces stress.

- **How to Dance for Fitness**:

1.    Choose your favorite music with an upbeat tempo.

2.      Start moving to the music with a variety of dance steps, such as side steps, shimmies, and twists.

3.      Let loose and have fun while staying active.

These cardiovascular exercises offer a range of options for beginners to elevate their heart rate, burn calories, and improve their overall fitness. Whether you prefer the simplicity of jumping jacks, the leg-strengthening benefits of high knees, the versatility of jumping rope, or the joyful experience of dancing, these exercises can be integrated into your home workout routine to boost your cardiovascular health.

# CHAPTER 6

# Strength Training

Strength training is a vital component of any well-rounded fitness routine. It helps build muscle, increase metabolism, and improve overall strength and endurance.

## 6.1 Bodyweight Exercises (Push-ups, Squats, Planks)

Bodyweight exercises are an excellent starting point for strength training, especially for beginners who may not have access to weights or equipment. Here's why bodyweight exercises are valuable and how to perform some basic ones:

**Benefits**:

- Builds functional strength using your body's own resistance.

- Requires no equipment, making it accessible for everyone.

- Engages multiple muscle groups and supports joint health.

- Can be easily modified to suit different fitness levels.

**How to Perform Bodyweight Exercises**:

- **Push-ups**:

  1. Start in a plank position with your hands shoulder-width apart.

  2. Lower your body by bending your elbows.

3.  Push back up to the
    starting position.

- **Squats**:

    1.  Stand with your feet
        shoulder-width apart.

    2.  Lower your body by
        bending your knees and
        pushing your hips back.

    3.  Return to the starting
        position by straightening
        your legs.

- **Planks**:

    1.  Get into a push-up
        position but with your
        weight on your forearms.

    2.  Keep your body in a
        straight line from head to
        heels, engaging your core
        muscles.

# 6.2 Using Household Items as Weights

Strength training doesn't always require expensive weights or equipment. Many household items can be used as improvised weights to add resistance to your workouts. Here's why this approach is beneficial and some examples of items you can use:

**Benefits**:

- Utilizes readily available items for resistance.

- Allows you to gradually increase the weight as you become stronger.

- Supports budget-friendly fitness options.

**Examples of Household Items as Weights**:

- Water bottles or milk jugs filled with water or sand.

- Backpack filled with books, canned goods, or other heavy items.

- Bags of rice or flour.

- Laundry detergent containers.

- Sturdy chairs for step-ups.

## 6.3 Resistance Band Workouts

Resistance bands are versatile and affordable tools that can be used for effective strength training at home. Here's why resistance bands are valuable and how to incorporate them into your workouts:

**Benefits**:

- Provide adjustable resistance for various exercises.

- Are portable and easy to store.

- Enhance muscle engagement and range of motion.

- Are suitable for a wide range of fitness levels.

**How to Use Resistance Bands**:

- **Bicep Curls**: Stand on the center of the band and curl the handles toward your shoulders.

- **Squats with Resistance**: Place the band under your feet and hold the handles on your shoulders while performing squats.

- **Lateral Leg Raises**: Attach the band to your ankles and perform leg lifts to the side for hip and thigh strengthening.

- **Pull-aparts**: Hold the band in front of you with both hands and pull it apart to work your upper back and shoulders.

Incorporating these strength training options into your home workout routine can help you build muscle, increase functional strength, and support overall fitness. Whether you prefer bodyweight exercises, household items as weights, or resistance bands, there are diverse and accessible ways for beginners to develop strength in the comfort of their own home.

# CHAPTER 7

# Flexibility and Mobility

Flexibility and mobility are essential components of overall fitness that often get overlooked. These aspects are critical for injury prevention, improving posture, and enhancing the quality of your daily movements.

## 7.1 Stretching Exercises

Stretching exercises play a crucial role in improving flexibility, reducing muscle tension, and enhancing joint range of motion. Here's why they're valuable and how to perform some basic stretching exercises:

**Benefits**:

- Increases flexibility, making everyday movements easier.

- Reduces the risk of muscle strains and injuries.

- Promotes relaxation and stress relief.

- Improves blood circulation and joint health.

**How to Perform Stretching Exercises**:

- **Hamstring Stretch**: Sit with one leg extended and the other bent so that the sole of your foot touches the inner thigh of the extended leg. Reach toward your toes to feel a stretch in the back of your thigh.

- **Chest Opener**: Stand with your feet shoulder-width apart, clasp your hands behind your back, and gently lift your arms to open up your chest.

- **Child's Pose**: Kneel on the floor, sit back on your heels, and extend your arms forward with your forehead touching the ground.

## 7.2 Yoga and Pilates for Beginners

Yoga and Pilates are holistic fitness practices that focus on flexibility, core strength, balance, and mindfulness. They are particularly beneficial for improving overall body mobility. Here's why they're valuable and how to get started as a beginner:

**Benefits**:

- Enhances flexibility and balance.

- Develops core strength and improves posture.

- Encourages relaxation and mental clarity.

- Can be adapted to various fitness levels.

**How to Start Yoga and Pilates**:

- **Online Resources**: There are many online videos and apps specifically designed for beginners. These resources guide you through poses and exercises at your own pace.

- **Yoga Mats**: Invest in a comfortable yoga or Pilates mat for better support and stability during your practice.

- **Beginner Classes**: If possible, consider attending beginner-friendly classes in your local area to receive guidance and support.

## 7.3 Foam Rolling Techniques

Foam rolling is a self-myofascial release technique that helps alleviate muscle tension and improve flexibility. Here's why foam rolling is beneficial and how to incorporate it into your routine:

**Benefits**:

- Relieves muscle tightness and knots.

- Enhances blood circulation and nutrient delivery to muscles.

- Reduces the risk of injury and improves range of motion.

- Promotes relaxation and recovery.

**How to Use a Foam Roller**:

- **Muscle Groups**: Focus on specific muscle groups. Roll slowly over the targeted area, applying moderate pressure.

- **Duration**: Spend 1-2 minutes on each muscle group, gradually working your way through your entire body.

- **Breathe**: Maintain relaxed breathing and try to breathe through any discomfort you may experience while rolling.

Incorporating these flexibility and mobility techniques into your home workout routine can help you move more freely, reduce the risk of injury, and enhance your overall physical well-being.

# CHAPTER 8

# Staying Motivated

Motivation is the driving force behind a successful fitness journey. It can be particularly challenging for beginners to maintain consistency and enthusiasm.

## 8.1 Setting and Tracking Goals

Setting clear and achievable goals is a fundamental step in staying motivated. Here's why goal setting is important and how to go about it:

**Benefits**:

- Provides a sense of purpose and direction.

- Breaks down your fitness
  journey into manageable steps.

- Keeps you accountable and
  focused.

- Offers a sense of achievement
  and progress.

**How to Set and Track Goals**:

- **Specific**: Define your goals
  with clarity. Instead of "I want
  to get fit," specify "I want to
  lose 10 pounds in three
  months."

- **Measurable**: Use quantifiable
  metrics to track your progress.
  This could be pounds lost,
  inches gained, or workout
  frequency.

- **Achievable**: Ensure that your
  goals are realistic and attainable

- based on your fitness level and resources.

- **Relevant**: Align your goals with your personal interests and long-term aspirations.

- **Time-bound**: Set a timeframe for your goals to create a sense of urgency and commitment.

- **Tracking Progress**: Use a workout journal, fitness app, or a simple calendar to track your progress and celebrate your achievements.

## 8.2 Finding Support and Accountability

Having a support system and accountability partners can significantly boost your motivation.

Here's why finding support is valuable and how to go about it:

**Benefits**:

- Provides encouragement and a sense of community.

- Offers a source of motivation and friendly competition.

- Increases the likelihood of sticking to your exercise routine.

- Helps you overcome challenges and setbacks.

**How to Find Support and Accountability**:

- **Workout Buddies**: Partner with a friend or family member who shares similar fitness goals. You can exercise together virtually or in person.

- **Online Communities**: Join fitness forums, social media groups, or online fitness classes where you can connect with like-minded individuals and receive support and advice.

- **Professional Guidance**: Consider working with a personal trainer or fitness coach who can provide expert advice, personalized workouts, and accountability.

- **Accountability Apps**: Use apps that track your workouts and progress while providing reminders and encouragement.

## 8.3 Overcoming Common Challenges

Recognizing and addressing common challenges that can deter your motivation is key to maintaining your momentum. Here's how to overcome some of these obstacles:

**Common Challenges**:

- **Lack of Time**: Incorporate short, effective workouts that fit your schedule.

- **Boredom**: Change up your routine regularly to keep things interesting.

- **Fatigue**: Listen to your body, get adequate rest, and avoid overtraining.

- **Lack of Results**: Adjust your goals and workout routine as needed. Plateaus are normal, and adaptation is part of the process.

- **Lack of Motivation**: Remind yourself of your "why" and the benefits of your fitness journey. Mix up your workouts to keep them exciting.

- **Injury or Health Concerns**: Prioritize safety and consult a healthcare professional or fitness expert if necessary.

# CHAPTER 9

# Safety and Injury Prevention

Safety and injury prevention are paramount when engaging in any exercise or fitness routine.

## 9.1 Listening to Your Body

Listening to your body is a fundamental aspect of safety and injury prevention in your exercise routine. Here's why it's crucial and how to go about it:

**Benefits**:

- Allows you to identify and respond to discomfort or pain.

- Helps you adjust your workouts to suit your current condition.

- Reduces the risk of overtraining and injuries.

- Promotes better mind-body awareness.

**How to Listen to Your Body**:

- **Pain vs. Discomfort**: Learn to differentiate between the discomfort associated with challenging workouts and actual pain. Pain is a sign that something is wrong, while discomfort can be part of the exercise process.

- **Rest and Recovery**: Recognize when your body needs rest and recovery. Overworking muscles without adequate rest can lead to injuries.

- **Modify as Needed**: Be willing to modify or skip exercises if they cause pain or discomfort. You can always return to them once you're stronger or more flexible.

- **Consult a Professional**: If you have concerns about pain or persistent discomfort, consult a healthcare professional or fitness expert.

## 9.2 Common Exercise Mistakes to Avoid

Avoiding common exercise mistakes is vital for injury prevention and effective workouts. Here are some of the most prevalent errors and how to steer clear of them:

**Common Exercise Mistakes:**

- **Poor Form**: Using improper form can strain muscles and joints. Ensure that you perform exercises with correct alignment and technique.

- **Overtraining**: Exercising too frequently or intensely without adequate rest can lead to overuse injuries and burnout. Incorporate rest days into your routine.

- **Skipping Warm-up and Cool-down**: Skipping warm-up and cool-down routines can increase the risk of injury. Always start with a warm-up and finish with a cool-down.

- **Neglecting Flexibility and Mobility**: Neglecting flexibility and mobility exercises can lead to reduced range of motion and muscle imbalances. Incorporate stretching and mobility work into your routine.

- **Inadequate Hydration and Nutrition**: Proper hydration and nutrition are essential for energy, performance, and recovery. Ensure you're well-hydrated and fuel your body with the nutrients it needs.

- **Ignoring Pain**: Pushing through pain or ignoring it is a common mistake. Pain is a signal that something is wrong. Stop and address the issue rather than continuing the exercise.

## 9.3 Dealing with Injuries

Despite best efforts, injuries can still occur. Knowing how to deal with injuries is essential for a safe and effective recovery:

**How to Deal with Injuries**:

- **RICE Method**: Rest, Ice, Compression, and Elevation can be effective for many minor injuries. Rest the injured area, apply ice, use compression (if applicable), and elevate it.

- **Seek Medical Attention**: If you suspect a severe or persistent injury, consult a healthcare professional for a proper diagnosis and treatment plan.

- **Rehabilitation and Modification**: Follow a

rehabilitation program as recommended by a healthcare provider. Modify your workouts as necessary to accommodate the injury.

- **Prevent Recurrence**: Focus on preventing a recurrence of the injury by addressing its underlying causes and weaknesses. Consult a physical therapist if needed.

# CHAPTER 10

# Nutrition and Recovery

Nutrition and recovery are integral aspects of any effective fitness regimen.

## 10.1 Fueling Your Body

Proper nutrition is the foundation for a successful home exercise routine. It provides the energy and nutrients your body needs for workouts and overall health. Here's why fueling your body is important and how to go about it:

**Benefits**:

- Sustains energy levels for effective workouts.

- Supports muscle repair and growth.

- Enhances overall health and well-being.

- Aids in weight management and body composition.

**How to Fuel Your Body**:

- **Balanced Diet**: Consume a well-balanced diet that includes a variety of whole foods like lean protein, complex carbohydrates, healthy fats, and a range of fruits and vegetables.

- **Timing**: Eat balanced meals and snacks throughout the day. Ensure that you have energy before workouts and replenish after exercising.

- **Hydration**: Stay well-hydrated. Dehydration can impair

exercise performance and overall well-being.

- **Pre-Workout Nutrition**: Consume a light meal or snack 1-2 hours before exercise to provide energy and prevent low blood sugar.

- **Post-Workout Nutrition**: Focus on protein and carbohydrates after your workout to support muscle recovery and replenish glycogen stores.

## 10.2 Post-Workout Nutrition

Post-workout nutrition is crucial for recovery and optimizing the benefits of your home exercise routine. Here's why it matters and how to approach it:

**Benefits**:

- Supports muscle recovery and growth.

- Replenishes glycogen stores.

- Aids in hydration and electrolyte balance.

- Reduces muscle soreness and fatigue.

**How to Approach Post-Workout Nutrition**:

- **Protein**: Consume a source of protein to aid muscle repair. Options include lean meats, dairy, plant-based proteins, or protein shakes.

- **Carbohydrates**: Replenish glycogen stores by consuming carbohydrates. Include whole grains, fruits, or starchy vegetables in your post-workout meal or snack.

- **Hydration**: Rehydrate with water or a sports drink, especially if you've had an intense workout and have lost a significant amount of sweat.

- **Timing**: Aim to eat or drink within 30 minutes to 2 hours after your workout to maximize recovery benefits.

- **Individual Needs**: Keep in mind that individual nutritional needs vary, so you may need to adjust based on your fitness goals and body's response.

## 10.3 Rest and Recovery

Rest and recovery are often underestimated but are essential for the success of your home exercise routine. Here's why they are crucial and how to prioritize them:

**Benefits**:

- Allows muscles to repair and grow.

- Reduces the risk of overtraining and injuries.

- Supports overall well-being and mental health.

- Improves workout performance and energy levels.

**How to Prioritize Rest and Recovery**:

- **Adequate Sleep**: Aim for 7-9 hours of quality sleep each night to allow your body to repair and recover.

- **Active Recovery**: Incorporate low-intensity activities like walking or stretching on rest days to promote blood flow and reduce muscle soreness.

- **Nutrition**: Ensure that your diet supports recovery with sufficient protein and nutrients.

- **Hydration**: Stay well-hydrated, as dehydration can impede the recovery process.

- **Stress Management**: Practice stress-reduction techniques like meditation, deep breathing, or yoga to support recovery and overall well-being.

- **Listen to Your Body**: If you feel fatigued or notice signs of overtraining, don't hesitate to take extra rest.

# CHAPTER 11

# Tracking Your Progress

Monitoring your progress is a vital component of your fitness journey. It provides motivation, helps you assess your improvements, and allows for necessary adjustments.

## 11.1 Keeping a Workout Journal

Keeping a workout journal is an effective way to document your fitness journey, track your accomplishments, and plan for future goals. Here's why maintaining a workout journal is important and how to do it:

**Benefits**:

- Offers a clear record of your workouts and progress.

- Helps you identify patterns, such as what exercises or routines work best for you.

- Provides motivation by visualizing how far you've come.

- Allows you to plan and adjust your future workouts.

**How to Keep a Workout Journal**:

- **Choose a Format**: You can use a physical notebook, a digital app, or even a simple spreadsheet to record your workouts.

- **Include Key Details**: Record details such as the date, exercises, sets, reps, weight lifted, duration, and notes about how you felt during the workout.

- **Set Goals**: Clearly define your fitness goals and document them in your journal. This helps you stay focused and measure your progress against your objectives.

- **Regular Updates**: Consistently update your journal after each workout to maintain an accurate record of your journey.

## 11.2 Measuring Success

Measuring success in your home exercise routine is essential for staying motivated and ensuring you're on the right track. Here's why it matters and how to measure your progress:

**Benefits**:

- Provides motivation and a sense of accomplishment.

- Helps you identify areas where you've improved.

- Assists in goal setting and refinement.

- Allows you to make data-driven adjustments to your workouts.

**How to Measure Your Success**:

- **Performance Metrics**: Track quantitative measures such as weight lifted, repetitions completed, time taken for specific exercises, or distance covered during cardio workouts.

- **Body Measurements**: Keep an eye on changes in your body measurements, like weight, body fat percentage, or circumference of specific body parts.

- **Fitness Tests**: Periodically conduct fitness tests related to your goals, such as endurance tests, flexibility assessments, or strength benchmarks.

- **Before-and-After Photos**: Take photographs before starting your fitness journey and at various points along the way to visually track changes in your physique.

- **Subjective Assessments**: Reflect on how you feel, your energy levels, and your overall well-being. These subjective assessments can be equally important in measuring success.

- **Goal Achievement**: Compare your progress against the goals you've set. If you're achieving your objectives, you're on the path to success.

www.ingramcontent.com/pod-product-compliance
Lightning Source LLC
Chambersburg PA
CBHW050840260726

48660CB00006B/2360